Best Natural Scrubs and Herbal Remedies For Your Health and Beauty

Table of content:

Book 1

**Body Scrubs: 35 Natural DIY Scrubs for Body and Face for Radiant and
Youthful Skin**.. 5

Introduction.. 6

Chapter 1 - What is a scrub? 7

Chapter 2 - The Recipes...17

Chapter 3 - Don't stop there... 34

Chapter 4 - Marketing and Selling 36

Conclusion 42

Book 2

Herbal Medicine: 30 Herbal Remedies to Heal Common Ailments 44

Introduction.. 45

Chapter 1 - An Introduction 46

Chapter 2 - The Structural System 62

Chapter 3 - The Circulatory System....................................... 67

Chapter 4 - Digestive System...71

Chapter 5 - Nervous System 74

Chapter 6 - The Glandular System 78

Chapter 7 - Keep Learning... 81

Conclusion... 82

Eva Warren

Body
Scrubs

35 Natural DIY Scrubs
For Body and Face
For Radiant and Youthful Skin

Body Scrubs:

35 Natural DIY Scrubs for Body and Face for Radiant and Youthful Skin

Introduction

Want to make your own scrubs

You have seen many scrubs in the store for your body and face. You have seen the results of using them, but the problem you would like to save money by making your own. You've looked all over the internet to find information on how to make scrubs on your own, but the flood of information is difficult to parse and find just what you are looking for in order to get started. In this book, I use my over twenty years of natural health experience to walk you through everything you will need to get started and eventually make your own. I will teach you the basics and leave you feeling like you can start making your own recipes and using them.

You're ready to get started...

By purchasing this book, you are ready to get started on a new way to take care of your skin and your body. This book will walk you through the steps and show you:

• What scrubs are and the different types.
• What essential oils are and how to use them
• The best ways to combine the essential oils
• Recipes with step-by-step instructions on how to make and store the scrubs

I will present the information in a fashion that is easy to understand without leaving you with more questions. I will walk you through every step of the process. So, if you're ready to get started, let's get to it.

Chapter 1 - What is a scrub?

We've seen all manner and types of scrubs to exfoliate and help to heal skin. Scrubs can smooth rough spots on elbows and knees. They can also help to lightly scrub off dead skin from the face and other areas well. It can also moisturize your skin as well.

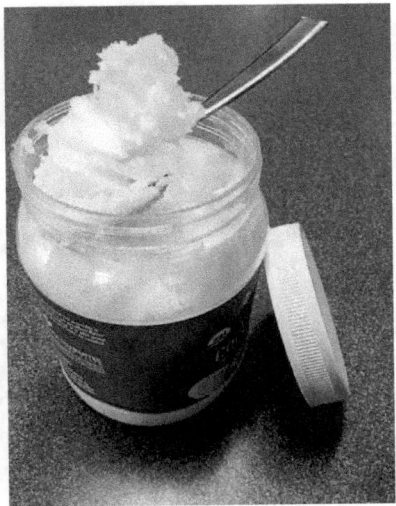

What you need...

There are a few simple things you will need to get started on your new hobby.

• Glass mixing bowls: You will need two of these to keep the dry ingredients separate from the wet ones until you are ready to mix them.

• Measuring cups: This is for measuring the sugar and other ingredients you will need.

• Wooden or glass spoons for mixing

• Airtight containers to store your scrubs

- Oils to mix into your scrubs

- Sugar, white or brown, preferably organic

- Essential oils

- Gloves to protect your hands while mixing

The oils

Before we get into the essential oils and safety, you need other oils, carrier oils to act as a base for the essential oil blends. Here is a list that you can use interchangeably or even mix together.

Coconut Oil

This oil is used more often than others when making scrubs because of the different fatty acids that tone and smooth skin.

It is solid at room temperature, which makes it good when placing the rub. It will melt when it comes in contact with the skin.

Olive Oil

This oil is also good for the skin because of its high concentration of vitamin E.

Almond Oil

Usually used for other preparations, I have found its very light, almost non-existent fragrance, makes it perfect for scrubs.

It is rich in protein and good for all types of skin. It also helps if you are suffering from dry and itchy and skins.

Apricot Kernel

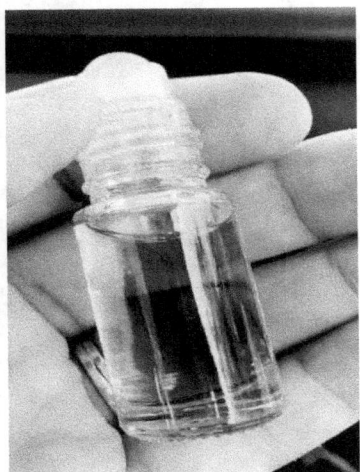

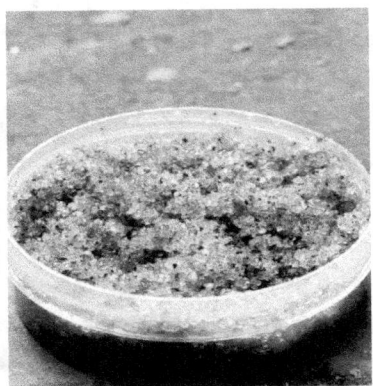

This is another light oil. It is used for sensitive skin. So, if you experience irritation from the other oils or are allergic to almonds, it is a good alternative because of its vitamin and mineral content.

Essential Oils

There are a list of essential oils you can use for your skin to help it look younger and healthier.

Cautions and Care

An essential oil is the most potent form of any plant; however, there are a few things you need to know about essential oils before you begin to use them.

1. Can cause contact dermatitis when used un-diluted. There are websites out there that will tell it is alright not to dilute the oils. This is false.

2. If you are not sure whether your skin will have a reaction to the use of certain essential oils, you can go to your nearest store that sells them and ask for a patch test. This will help you determine which essential oils will be alright for you to use.

3. Store the essential oils in a cool, dry place. Many essential oils are very light and will evaporate when exposed to heat.

4. Store your scrubs in tightly lidded dark glass containers to prevent light from entering and possibly heating up the mixture.

5. Scrubs have the same shelf life as the sugar you used to make them. It is best not to keep them longer than that. For maximum potency, use them after letting sit overnight in the container.

6. Do not apply scrubs to cracked, raw skin or open wounds. It will irritate the area to which it is applied.

The listc v

Bergamot, *Citrus bergamia*
This one is good for treating cold sores as well as acne, and greasy skin.

Cedarwood, Texas, *Juniperus ashei*
This is the first of two types of Cedarwood that are used for skin issues. This help with oily skin, it also helps with acne, eczema, psoriasis.

Cedarwood, Virginian, *Juniperus virginiana*
This essential oil is also good for the same things of its relative. The difference is, being a different genus, it can be gentler than the Texas version.

Chamomile, Roman, *Chamaemelum nobile*
This is an especially good essential oil for acne, eczema, light rashes, dermatitis, and inflammations.

Clary Sage, *salvia sclarea*
This is an essential oil that is good for regulating oily skin, and also helping to reduce swelling and fight acne. It's good for wrinkles, too.

Clove Bud, *Syzygium armaticum*
This is good for stubborn acne.

Galbanum, *Ferula galbaniflua*
This helps to heal scar tissue, tones skin, wrinkles as well as acne.

Geranium, *Pelargonium graveolens*
This essential oil is excellent for speeding the healing of broken capillaries, acne, burns, helps to unclog pores, and balances an oily complexion.

Grapefruit, *Citrus x paradisi*

This essential oil helps to tone and reduce sagging in skin and skin. It helps to unclog pore and regulate skin. It is also good for acne.

Helichrysum, *Helichrysum angutifolium*

This essential oil can help with inflammations of the skin caused by rosacea and puffiness around the eyes, chin and other problem areas. It has also been used to help treat acne, dermatitis, eczema, and age spots and blemishes for pinched zits.

Juniper, *Juniperus communis*

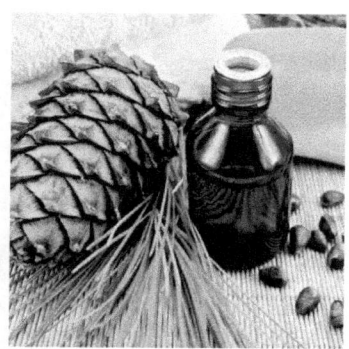

This essential oil is used to help treat acne breakouts and existing pimples. It has also been used to help treat skin conditions such as dermatitis and rosacea. It is also a skin toner.

Lavender, *Lavendula angustifolia*

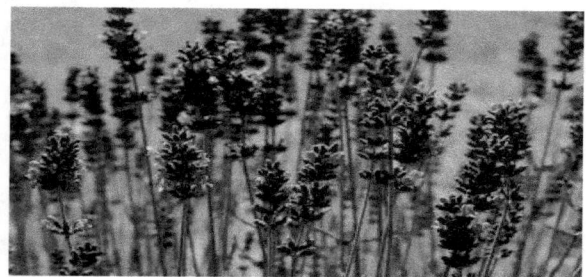

This is an all-around essential oil for promoting healthy skin. It helps to reduce blemishes and scarring and helps to speed healing of acne that has been pinched. It also has antiseptic properties.

Lime, *Citrus aurantifolia*
This is another good one for spots in the skin, warts, greasy skin, and acne.

Myrtle, *Myrtus communis*
This essential oil is highly recommended for treating oily skin and it helps to open pours for a deeper cleansing.

Naouli, *Melaluca viridiflora*
This is another oil that is good for treating oily skin and all types of acne.

Palmarosa, *Cymbopogon martinii var. martinii*
Another essential oil that helps to reduce scarring and wrinkles, it is also recommended for acne, dry skin conditions. It also helps to moisturize the skin.

Patchouli, *Pogostemon cablin*
This is essential is used for a very wide array of skin conditions. Not only does it treat acne, it also helps with rosacea, dermatitis, eczema, fungal infections, oily skin, helps to shrink open pores, and wrinkles.

Peppermint, *Mentha piperita*
This essential oil has antiseptic properties. It is also good for treating acne.

Rosemary, *Rosmarinus officinalis*
This is one that is not recommended if you have hypertension as it can raise the blood pressure. It is used mainly for acne, dermatitis, and eczema.

Rosewood, *Aniba rosaeodora*
This essential oil helps to bring combination complexions into balance. It is also good for general, everyday skin care. It is good for regular and sensitive skin.

Sandalwood, *Santalum album*

Helps to regulate greasy skin and can be an efficient moisturizer. This is also good for acne.

Tea Tree, *Melaluca Alternifolia*

Because of its aroma, it is used in small does, but it is a potent skin toner and treatment for acne. It also helps to treat oily skin.

There are more essential oils than this on the market, but these are the ones I highly recommend for scrubs.

Thyme, *Thymus Vulgaris*

Like many others, it helps to regulate oily skin and fight acne. Thyme should be avoided when pregnant. Overuse can lead to sensitivity of the essential oil.

Vetiver, *Vetiveria zizanioe*

This essential oil helps to combat acne and oily skin.

Violet, *Viola odorata*

Violet essential oil helps to refine pours, smooth out eczema, and treat acne.

Yarrow, *Achillea millefolium*

This essential oil helps to tone the skin as well as treat skin conditions like eczema, inflammations, and rashes. It also helps to treat acne.

Ylang Ylang, *Canaga odorata var. genuina*

This is another essential oil for general skin care. It helps with irritated and inflamed skin. Also helps treat acne, and oily skin.

Combining Essential Oils

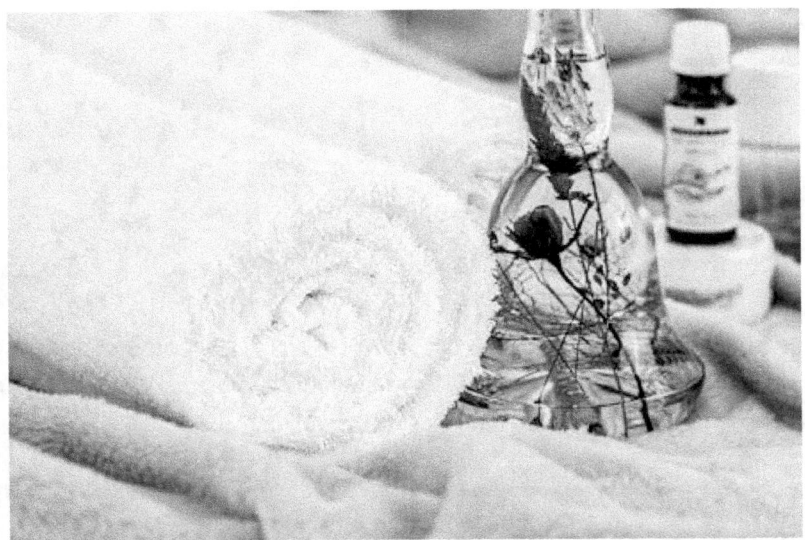

There are three types of essential oils:

Light
Medium,
And heavy.

These are usually known as "notes". When combining them, you will generally use more of the light and medium than you would the heavy. Making blends is usually in small batches, one tablespoon at a time. Here is a standard blend measure:

1 tbsp+6 drops of essential oil.

Now, obviously making scrubs, especially in large batches, would mean you're using more than one tablespoon in most cases. So, here is another guide.

Base recipe for Sugar scrubs:

1/2 cup sugar, white or brown

1/2 cup oil

50 Drops essential oil blend

• Blend the oils first.

• Stir the sugar into the oil blend.

Instructions for use:

Place thins layer of the scrub on the face, elbows, knees, or any non-sensitive part of the body. Scrub the area in small circles. Rinse with warm water and soap.

Now, that we've got the basics out of the way. Let's get on with the recipes.

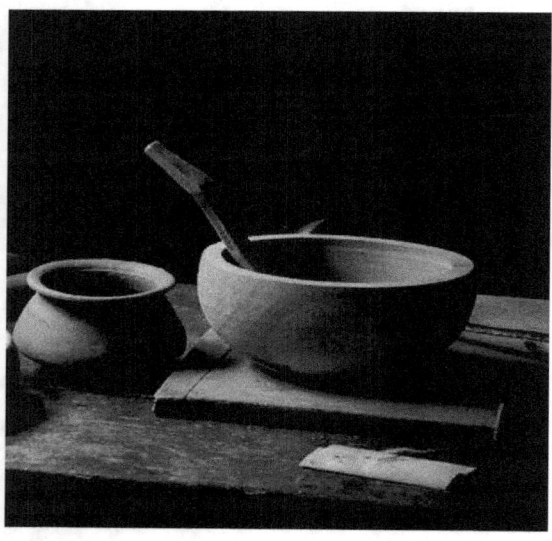

Chapter 2 - The Recipes

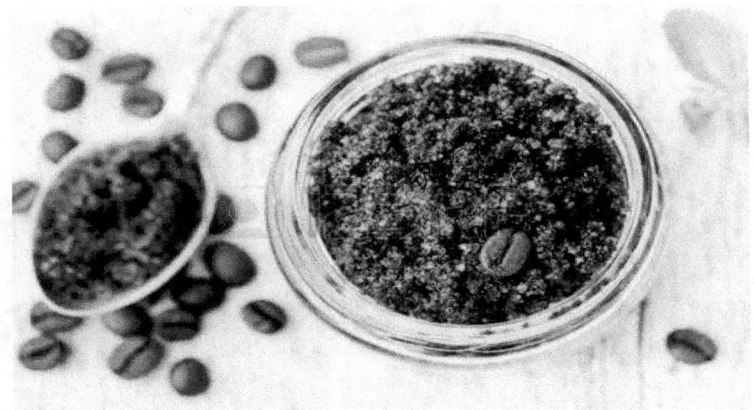

1. Oily Skin I

1/4 Cup Coconut Oil

1/4 Cup Almond Oil

20 Drops Lavender Essential Oil

10 Drops Tea Tree Essential Oil

10 Drops Texas Cedarwood Essential Oil

10 Drops Clary Sage Essential Oil

2. Oily Skin II

1/4 Cup Almond Oil

1/4 Cup Olive Oil

20 Drops Geranium Essential Oil

10 Drops Juniper Essential Oil

10 Drops Palmarosa Essential Oil

10 Drops Roman Chamomile Essential Oil

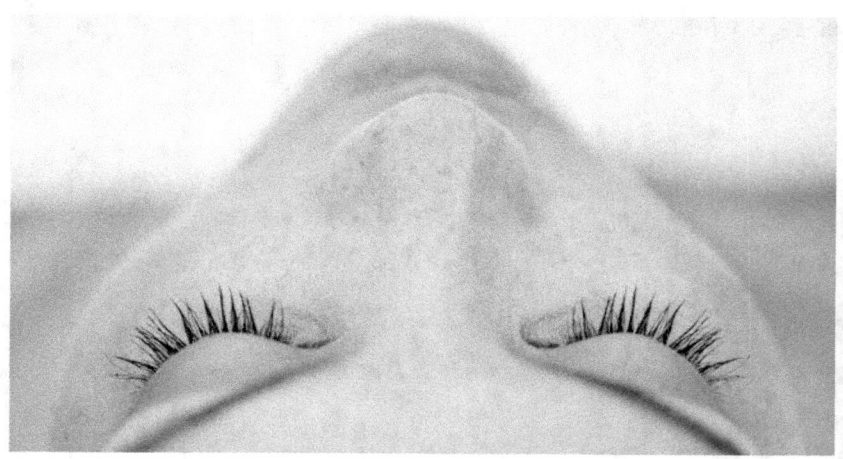

No doubt many of you have seen me type both "greasy" and "oily skin". There is a slight difference between the two. Oily skin tends to maintain a sheen on your face which is steady throughout the day, making you constantly check your makeup to cover those "shiny spots". Greasy skin is a more severe form of oily skin. Greasy skin produces more oils, making it impossible to go through a day and not have to wash your face to get rid of the excess oils.

There are ways of combatting oily/greasy skin besides washing your face and using scrubs:

1. Moisturize your skin. I know this may seem like you are adding oils to an already oily situation, but a nice and light moisturizer can prevent your skin from pulling in or producing too much oil to keep itself from drying out.

2. Keep a food diary. Even though many may say what you eat will not affect your skin, not all body chemistry is the same. One person can eat as much chocolate as they want and never have a skin problem while another, figuratively, breaks out just by looking at the confection.

3. Don't overdo it with washing your face. Keeping you face clean is a good idea, but if you are washing your face more than twice a day, you may be washing it too much. Your skin needs to produce some natural oils to maintain a pH balance, and when you are constantly washing your skin, you're forcing it to over compensate.

3. Greasy skin I

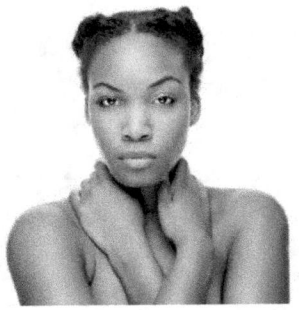

1/2 Cups Almond Oil
20 Drops Bergamot Essential Oil
10 Drops Lime Essential Oil
5 Drops Sandalwood Essential Oil
15 Drops Myrtle Essential Oil
10 Drops Virginia Cedarwood Essential Oil

4. Greasy Skin II

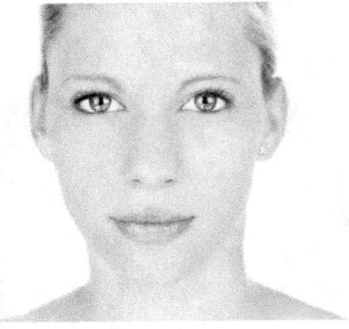

1/2 Cup Apricot Oil
20 Drops Lime Essential Oil
10 Drops Peppermint Essential Oil
10 Drops Patchouli Essential Oil
10 Drops Rosewood Essential Oil

5. Skin Toner

1/2 Cup Coconut Oil
20 Drops Grapefruit Essential oil
10 Drops Violet Essential Oil
10 Drops Juniper Essential Oil
10 Drops Rosewood Patchouli Essential Oil

6. Sensitive Skin Toner

1/4 Cup Almond Oil
1/4 Cup Olive Oil
20 Drops Lavender Essential Oil
10 Drops Rosewood Essential Oil
10 Drops Violet Essential Oil
10 Drops Ylang Ylang Essential Oil

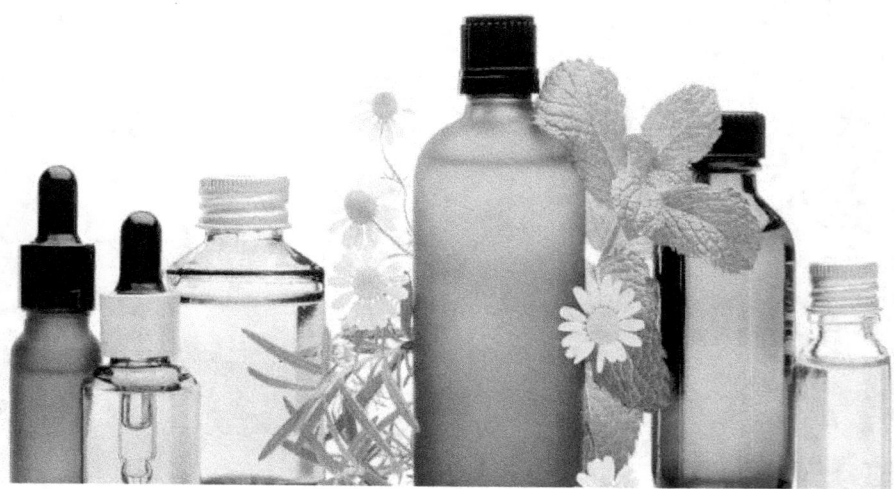

7. Dry Skin I

1/4 Cup Olive Oil
1/4 Coconut Oil
20 Drops Palmarosa Essential Oil
15 Drops Lavender Essential Oil
15 Drops Peppermint Essential Oil

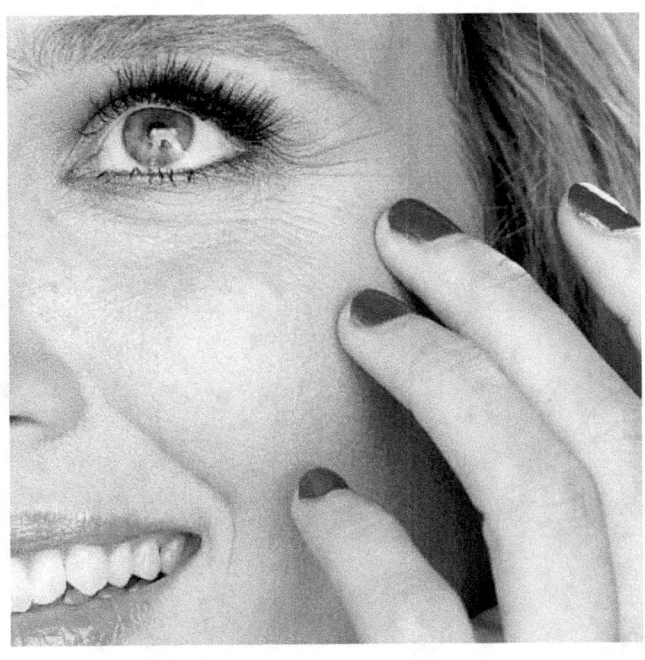

8. Dry Skin II

1/2 Cup Coconut Oil
15 Drops Rosewood Essential Oil
15 Drops Naouli Essential Oil
10 Drops Patchouli Essential Oil
10 Drops Vetiver Essential Oil

9. Toning I

1/4 Cup Coconut Oil
1/4 Cup Apricot Oil
15 Drops Grapefruit Essential Oil
15 Drops Juniper Essential Oil
10 Drops Virginia Cedarwood Essential Oil
10 Drops Sandalwood Essential Oil

10. Toning II

1/2 Coconut Oil
20 Drops Grapefruit Essential Oil
15 Drops Lavender Essential Oil
15 Drops Galbanum Essential Oil

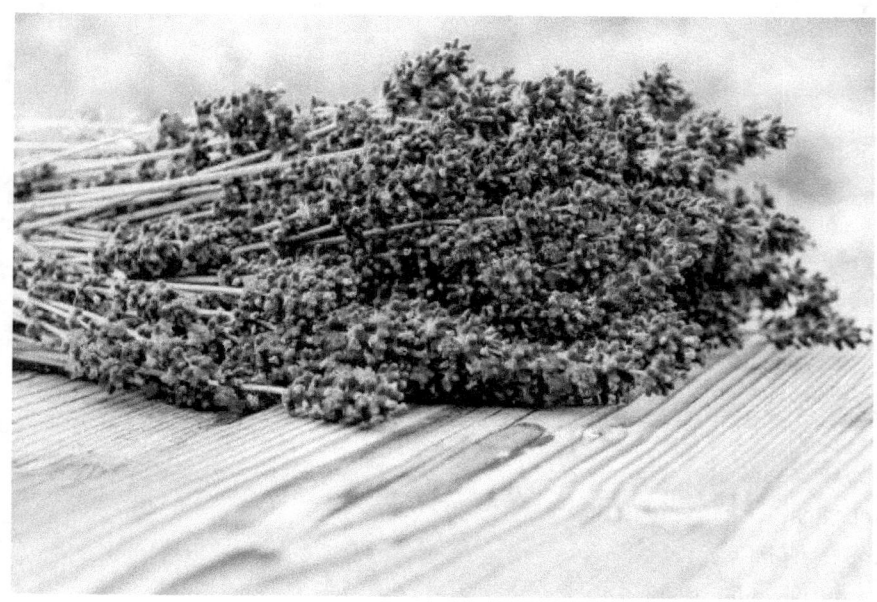

11. Wrinkle Scrub

1/4 Cup Coffee dry coffee grounds
1/4 Cup Cacao Ground
1/2 Cup Coconut Oil
20 Drops Lavender Essential Oil
10 Drops Clary Sage Essential Oil
10 Drops Palmarosa
10 Drops Grapefruit

12. Toning Scrub III

1/2 Cup Coffee Grounds
1/2 Cup Coconut Oil
20 Drops Grapefruit Essential Oil
15 Drops Roman Chamomile Essential Oil
15 Drops Peppermint Essential Oil

13. Soothing I

1/4 Cup Olive Oil
1/4 Cup Almond Oil
20 Drops Geranium Essential Oil
15 Drops Galbanum Essential Oil
15 Drops Vetiver Essential Oil

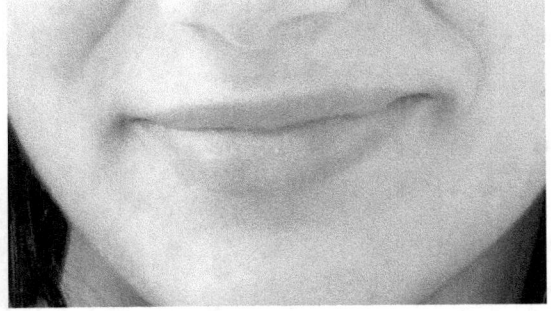

14. Soothing II

1/4 Cup Coconut Oil
1/4 Cup Almond Oil
15 Drops Violet
15 Drops Ylang Ylang
10 Drops Myrtle Essential Oil
10 Drops Rosewood Essential Oil

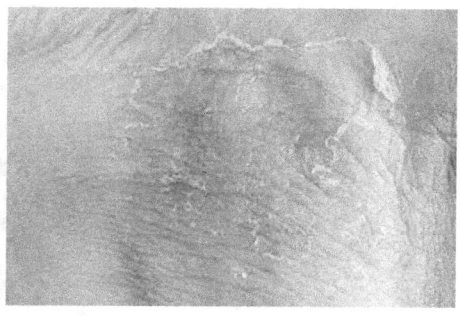

15. Eczema I

(Don't rub into broken skin)
1/2 Cup Coconut Oil
20 Drops Lavender Essential Oil
15 Drops Rosewood Essential Oil
5 Drops Sandalwood Oil
10 Drops Patchouli Essential Oil

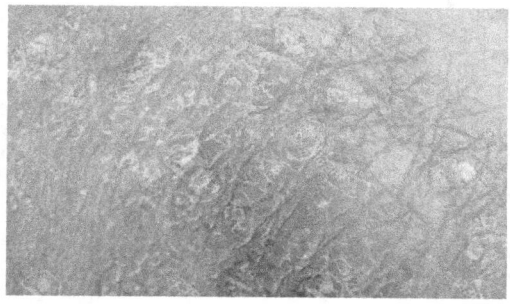

16. Eczema II

(Don't rub on broken skin)
1/2 Almond Oil
15 Drops Chamomile Essential Oil
15 Drops Lavender Essential Oil
10 Drops Violet Essential Oil
10 Drops Juniper Essential Oil

17. General Use I

1/2 Cup Olive Oil
10 Drops Lavender Essential Oil
10 Drops Grapefruit Essential Oil
10 Drops Rosewood Essential Oil
10 Drops Chamomile Essential Oil
10 Drops Myrtle Essential Oil

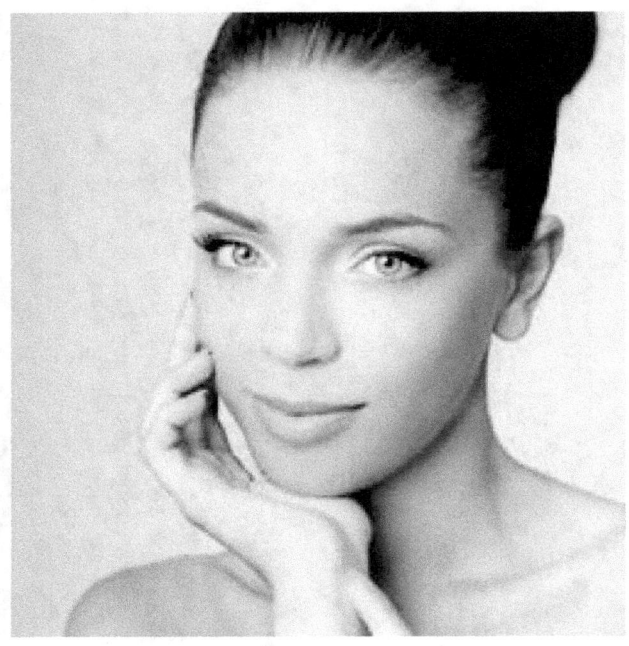

18. General Use II

1/2 Cup Coconut Oil
15 Drops Lavender Essential Oil
10 Drops Peppermint Essential Oil
10 Drops Palmarosa Essential Oil
5 Drops Clove Essential Oil
10 Drops Galbanum Essential Oil

19. Refining I

1/8 Cup Olive Oil
1/8 Cup Coconut Oil
1/4 Cup Almond Oil
15 Drops of Geranuim Essential Oil
10 Drops of Patchouli Essential oil
15 Drops of Lime Essential Oil
10 Drops Peppermint Essential Oil

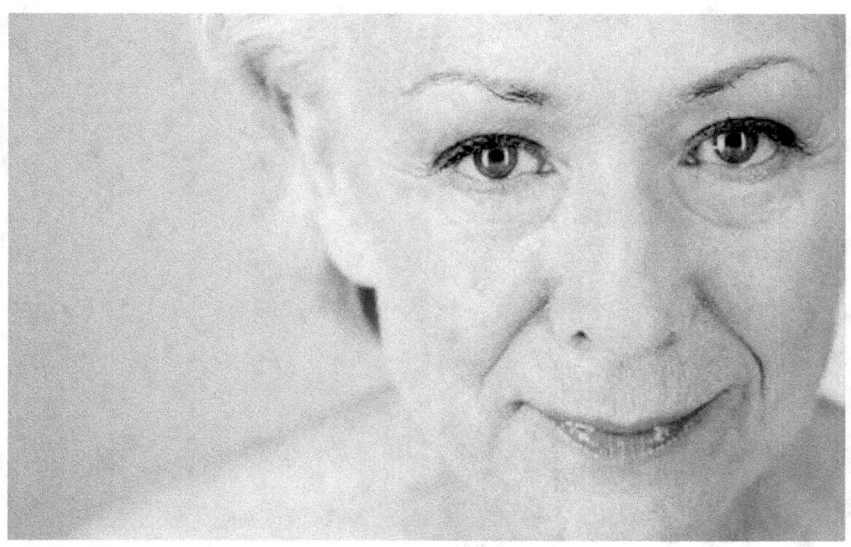

20. Refining II Mature Skin

This one is recommended for older skin.
1/4 Cup Olive Oil
1/4 Cup Coconut Oil
20 Drops of Violet Essential Oil
15 Drops of Palmarosa Essential Oil
10 Drops Vetiver Essential Oil
5 Drops Myrrh Essential Oil (refines and smooths skin for older complexions)

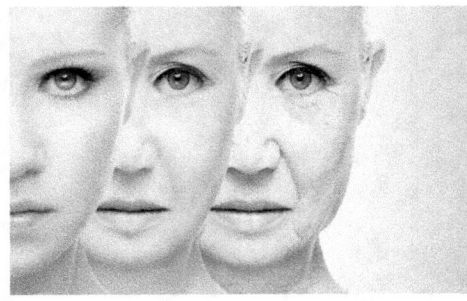

21. Toning for Mature Skin

1/2 Cup Olive Oil
15 Drops Myrtle Essential Oil
15 Drops Naouli Essential Oil
10 Drops Peppermint Essential Oil
10 Drops Grapefruit Essential Oil

22. General Care for Mature Skin

1/2 Cup Coconut Oil
15 Drops Lavender Essential Oil
15 Drops Rosewood Essential Oil
10 Drops Violet Essential Oil
10 Drops Ylang Ylang Essential Oil

23. Oily Mature Skin

1/2 Cup Almond Oil
15 Drops Naouli Essential Oil
10 Drops Bergamot Essential Oil
15 Drops Violet Essential Oil
10 Drops Helichrysum Essential Oil

24. Disinfectant Scrub I

1/2 Cup Coconut Oil
20 Drops Lavender Essential Oil
10 Drops Peppermint Oil
10 Drops Tea Tree Oil
10 Drops Lime Essential Oil

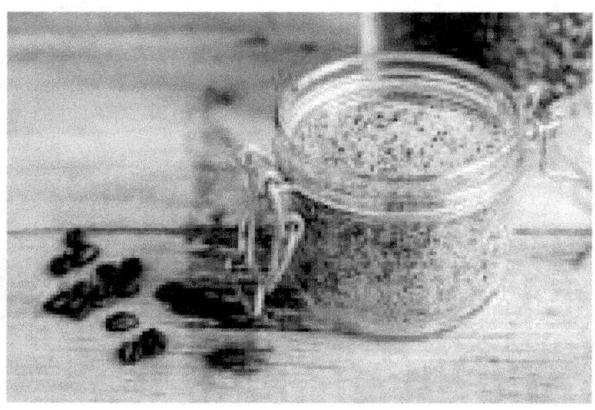

25. Disinfectant and Toning

1/2 Cup Coconut Oil
20 Drops Bergamot Essential Oil
10 Drops Tea Tree Oil
10 Drops Naouli Essential Oil
10 Drops Geranium Essential Oil

26. Disinfectant and Balancing

1/4 Cup Almond Oil
1/4 Cup Coconut Oil
15 Drops Myrtle Essential Oil
15 Drops Patchouli Essential Oil
10 Drops Peppermint Essential Oil
10 Drops Grapefruit Essential Oil

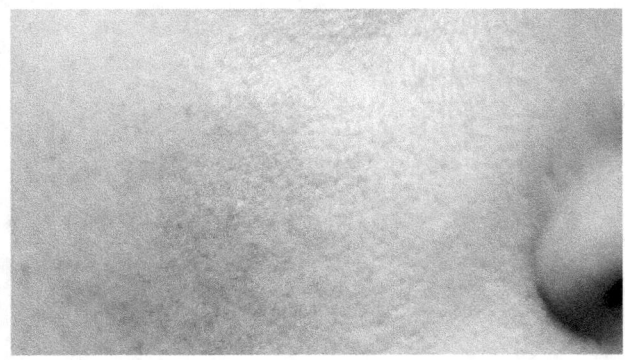

27. Rosacea I

(Don't rub on broken skin or weeping spots)
1/2 Cups Coconut Oil
15 Drops Lavender Essential Oil
15 Drops Rosewood Essential Oil

10 Drops Patchouli Essential Oil
10 Drops Myrtle Essential Oil

28. Rosacea II

1/2 Cup Olive Oil
15 Drops Palmarosa Essential Oil
15 Drops Galbanum Essential Oil
10 Drops Chamomile Essential Oil
10 Drops Tea Tree Essential Oil

29. Exfoliating and Refining I

1/4 Cup roughly ground Coffee grounds
1/4 Cup roughly ground Brown Sugar
1/2 Cup Coconut Oil
15 Drops Grapefruit Essential Oil
15 Drops Peppermint Essential Oil
10 Drops Geranium Essential Oil
10 Drops Helichrysum Essential Oil

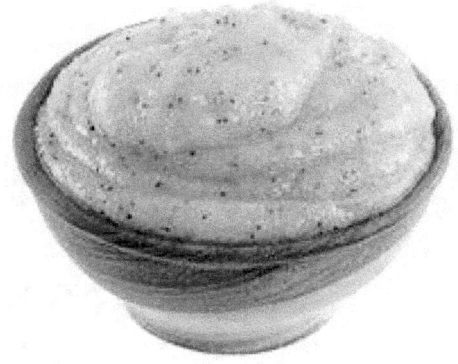

30. Exfoliating and Refining II

1/4 Cup roughly ground Coffee grounds
1/4 Cup roughly ground Brown Sugar
1/2 Cup Coconut Oil
20 Drops Galbanum Essential Oil
10 Drops Pathchouli Essential Oil
10 Drops Grapefruit Essential Oil
10 Drops Lime Essential Oil

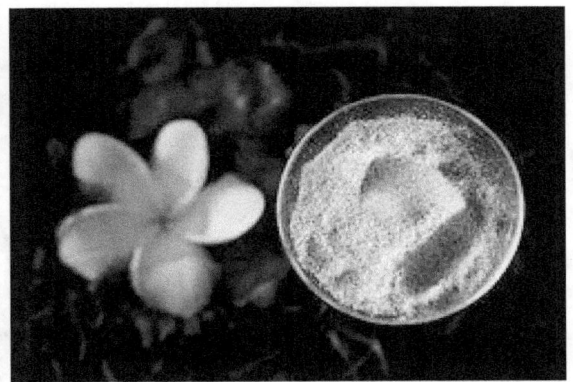

31. Soothing for Mature Skin

1/2 Cup of Coconut Oil
20 Drops of Lavender Essential Oil
15 Drops Palmarosa Essential Oil
15 Drops Rosewood Essential Oil

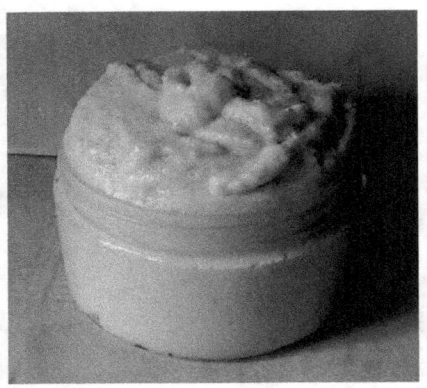

32. Dry Skin for Mature Complexion

1/2 Cup of Olive Oil
15 Drops Chamomile Essential Oil
15 Drops Palmarosa Essential Oil
10 Drops Peppermint Essential Oil
10 Drops Ylang Ylang Essentail Oil

33. Everyday Scrub

1/2 Cup Coconut Oil
10 Drops Chamomile Essential Oil
10 Drops Peppermint Essential Oil
10 Drops Rosewood Essential Oil
10 Drops Grapefruit Essential Oil
10 Drops Palmarosa Essential Oil

34. Mocha Scrub

1/4 Cup Ground Cacao
1/4 Cup Coffee Grinds
1/2 Cup Coconut Oil
15 Drops Rosewood Essential Oil
15 Drops Peppermint Essential Oil
10 Drops Vetiver Essential Oil
10 Drops Bergamot Essential Oil

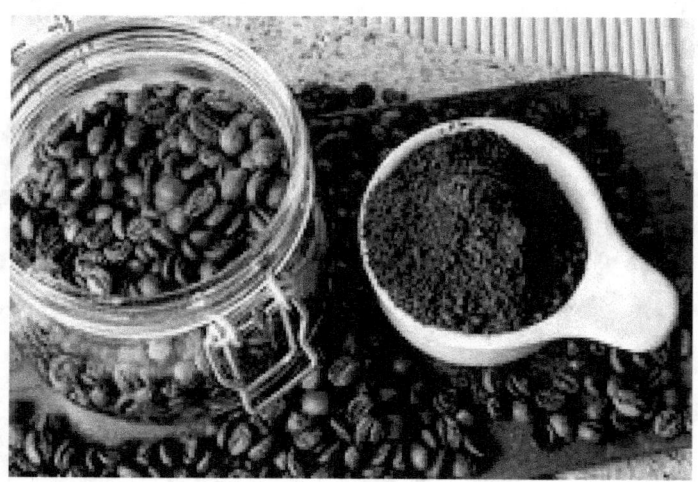

35. Mocha Scrub II

1/4 Cup Ground Cacao
1/4 Cup Coffee Grinds
1/2 Cup Coconut Oil
20 Drops Grapefruit Essential Oil
15 Drops Palmarosa Essential Oil
15 Drops Myrtle Essential Oil

Chapter 3 - Don't stop there...

This is just the start of your hobby. To get a better understanding of essential oils and aromatherapy, join forums where people of like mind share tips, tricks, and knowledge of this most rewarding hobby.

Branch out. Don't just make scrubs. There are so many things you can do with essential oils, and you're ready to look into it. You can make

• Mineral baths
--These can be made of either salts or oatmeal and is good for reducing muscle pains and swelling and softens the skin.

• Facial masks
--Essential oils with their base oils can be mixed with clay powders to tone and cleanse the face.

• Massage oils
--You can combine different essentials with their base oils loosen tight muscles and relax the body.

• Homemade soap
--You can add essential oils to homemade soap to give them an extra kick to cleanse and tone the skin.

• Shampoo Additives
--You can add essential oils to your favorite shampoo to make your hair healthier

• Lotions
--You can either by base lotion or add essential oils to your existing lotion to boost its effectiveness

There are more oils out there

There are over 80 essential oils on the market which can be used for a multitude of purposes and to help treat illnesses.

Resources

There are Ebooks and books you can get at books stores to expand your knowledge on aromatherapy. You can also find forums online with knowledgeable people who can give you advice and recipes. There are websites dedicated to essentials and their uses.

Chapter 4 - Marketing and Selling

When you are comfortable with making your own original recipes and even mixing the ones in the previous chapter, you may wonder if you can break into packaging and selling your own. You can, but there are a few things you will need to get your name out there.

Brand Name

This should be catchy and also tell your potential customers what you are selling. It should be easy to remember and find on the internet.

Labels and Packaging

There are websites out there which can help you design a logo and place the logo on your packaging. You can find the best services when you shop around online.
Look up regulations in your area to see what the requirements are for the ingredients on the label and if you need a disclaimer.

Mixing and Testing

It takes months to formulate, test, and make sure your recipes are safe and effective. You can test the recipes on yourself and your friends and family, if they are willing. Once you have a good base of recipes that work, you are ready to start marketing your products.

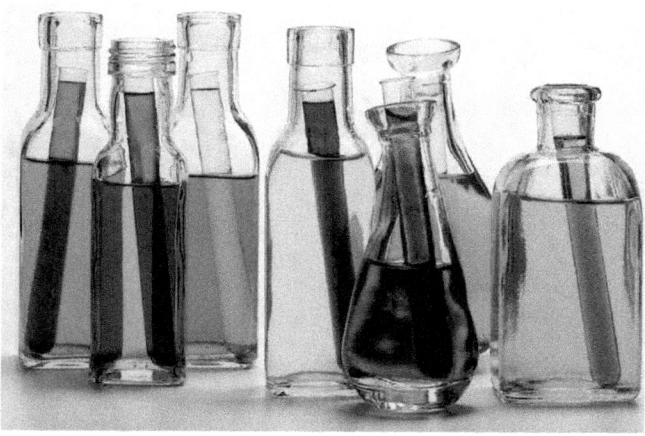

Marketing

No matter what your product is, you have to sell yourself first. You do this by showing the knowledge you have gained through the process. You then build a rapport with your potential customers before you introduce you product line.

Blog

Blogs are a wonderful way to start getting your name out there and showing what you know about essential oils and aromatherapy. Categorized correctly, it makes it easier for you customer base to find in the information. You can also include the process you go through to make your products. As you introduce your products, you can make a blog post with the ingredients and how they work. This will help your customers make a more informed decision.

Social Media

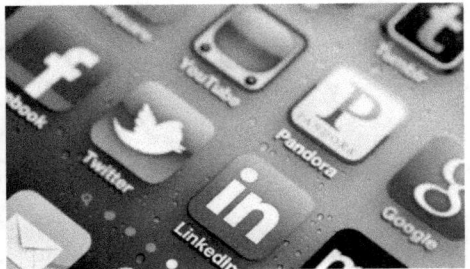

This is a free and effective way to get your name out there. Here are a few things platforms you can use to market your products:

Facebook

Even though they keep changing their algorithm, you can still get your name out there in two ways:

1. Fan Page: With a fan page, you can announce new products, upcoming blog posts and even post info-graphics and small info-memes to keep your customers in the know.

2. Groups: You can start your own group and advertise in it and invite people to join. You can also use this as an online forum to interact further with your customers.

Twitter

You can put small tips and tricks in 140 characters for your customers that like to get quick bursts of information. You can also post info memes and share your blog links here, too.

Instagram

This is where you can really show off your product. You can display product pictures, before and after pictures, and even post informational pictures for your customers to look at and comment on.

Snapchat

You can post short video announcements for new products and answer questions. You can also make sale announcements, too.

YouTube

This may not be an obvious choice for marketing, but making a video on how you make your products will provide a behind-the-scenes way for your customers to find out how products are made. You can also make short informational videos to share on other platforms.

Social Media Marketing Tips

To be effective, there are certain things you need to know about navigating social media:

1. It's social media, not commercial media
--This may sound counter-productive, but sharing little tidbits of your day and what are up to makes you more personable to your customer base. Make about 30% of your media posts about your day.

2. Images attract attention

--Infographics, memes, and collages of your products will draw a customer's eyes to your page and posts. It will increase organic reach and interaction.

3. Interact on other like pages

--Search for other people with interests like yours to engage with and start conversations. Join groups and forums to get your name out there and show your knowledge.

4. Use dashboards

--Use tools like Hootsuite and Buffer to keep all of your social media in one place. These dashboards will let you share your posts over all media without having to go to each one individually. Hootsuite even has tools you can use to receive notifications when someone mentions your name or products without a hashtag.

6. Know your hashtags

7.

--Rite tag is the perfect for making sure your tweets and google+ plus posts will have the best hashtags for the most reach.

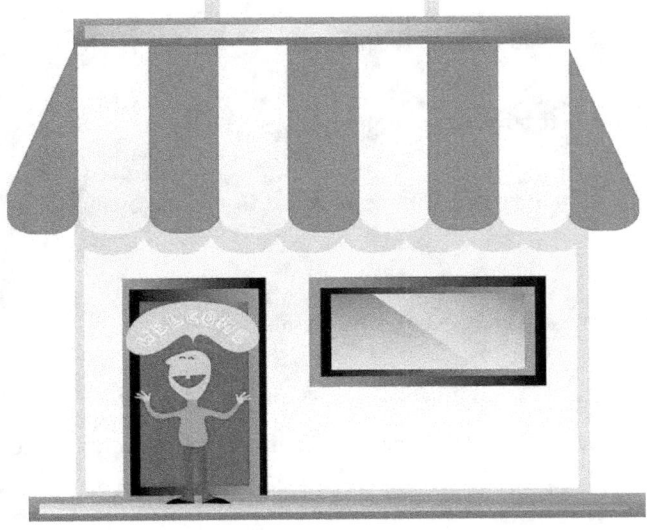

Pricing

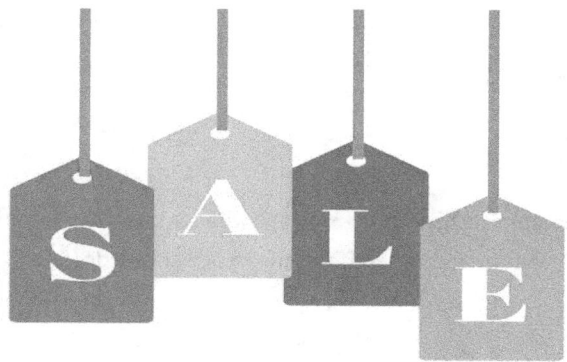

Besides getting the recipes right, the next hardest thing is figuring out how to price your products. Here is what needs to be factored into your final price:

1.   Your labels and packaging,

2.   Shipping,

3.   The individual products you mix in your products,

4.   The time is takes you to formulate and test the product,

5.   Any marketing tools you use to advertise your products,

6.   A portion of your home's mortgage or rent appropriate to the space you use to make your products divided by the number of products you make in a month,

7.   A percentage of the utilities used in the part of your residence,

8.   Finally, the percentage that will constitute your profit.
There are forums online you can go to and ask for more information and formulas to price your products.

Offline Marketing

There are stores out there which are operated by the owners. Before you approach them there are a few things you need to do:

1. Call and introduce yourself and your business. Be professional and polite. Explain the type of products you make and if they would be interested in trying samples. If they say yes, make small samples of the products and have a presentation ready.

2. Your presentation should be quick, concise and informative. It should include how long it would take for you to fill an order for their store and how much stock you have ready to fill that order.

3. Have a cost price for your products. This price should be 10%-20% of the wholesale price (the price of the materials you use).

Open air Markets

You can contact local and out-of-state venues to sell your items.

1. Many cities across the U.S. have monthly markets which will let you set up a booth and sell your products.

2. You can go to Pow-wows to sell your products as well. Native American Pow-wows will also let you set up tents to sell your wares

3. There are also natural health conventions you can register and sell your products.

If you are planning to do any of these, prepare to make more than one trip to these venues. You have to establish a presence and connect with other vendors and venue-goers. Planning on going to several of these each year will expose you to more customers and even customers you've met online will probably be at these events. This will give you a chance to meet them.

Conclusion

I hope this book served you well. I hope the information contained within answered questions and got your creative juices flowing. Never stop making new things. See you next book!

HERBAL MEDICINE:

30

Herbal Remedies to Heal Common Ailments

Olivia Palmer

Herbal Medicine:

30 Herbal Remedies to Heal Common Ailments

Introduction

You want to take control of your health.

The problem is there is too much information out there to sift through, and it's getting hard to tell the difference between fake remedies and proven ones. You looked up information online, in books, and have even asked owners and managers of health foods stores only to find you still have questions and wonder if the information is accurate. Wait no longer! I wrote this book with those concerns in mind. I have taken the time to sort through all the information and combed through studies to find the most relevant information on herbal medicine. I also walk you through what you need to make your own remedies and how long they keep before you have to make them again. I even include any possible side-effects and interactions with prescription drugs. What are you waiting for?

Chapter 1 - An Introduction

Herbalism has been around for millennia. It started in ancient China by trial and error. This meant they tried different plants to test their effects and rushed to find an antidote when they would accidentally ingest a poison. Though this doesn't seem like the smartest to document herbs and their uses, it eventually developed into what Asia knows as Traditional Chinese Medicine, which they practice to this day. India founded and still practices Ayurdeva, and Europe has an herbal pharmacology. In this day age, many mainstream physicians will work with people who have chosen to take herbal supplements.

The philosophy behind herbalism is approaching illness from a holistic method, meaning the whole body is looked at and not just the illness. By treating the body, mind, and spirit as well as the illness as one, the body will generally heal faster. This will also mean changes to lifestyle, diet, and how you mentally feel while you are ill. When symptoms are addressed by a holistic physician, they will be treated in the opposite order in which they manifested. Holistic medicine is about finding the root cause of the illness, not just treating symptoms.

This is a concern for many who delve into taking herbal supplements or taking herbal remedies for the first time. There are a few things to keep in mind.

Your body knows what you need. Learn to listen to it.

Your body know what's best for you. If you are taking an herbal supplement at start having reactions like headaches, indigestion, or other things along those lines, this is your body's way of telling you it doesn't need it.

If you are allergic to one plant in the family, be careful with other in the same genus/species.

Ragweed and Chamomile are related. This means if you are allergic to the weed, you may have reactions to the herb. Spend time looking to the herb you are interested in taking to make sure you are not allergic to its relatives.

If you are taking prescriptions for a medical condition, avoid herbs that work against it or will boost its potency.

An example of this would be Gingko Biloba, which has been proven to help improve memory. It is also a blood thinner. It is not recommended for you to take this herb if you are on medication to either thin the blood or reduce plaque deposits in your blood vessels. This also goes for beta blocker prescriptions and any herbals that are recommended for migraines or anti-depressants.

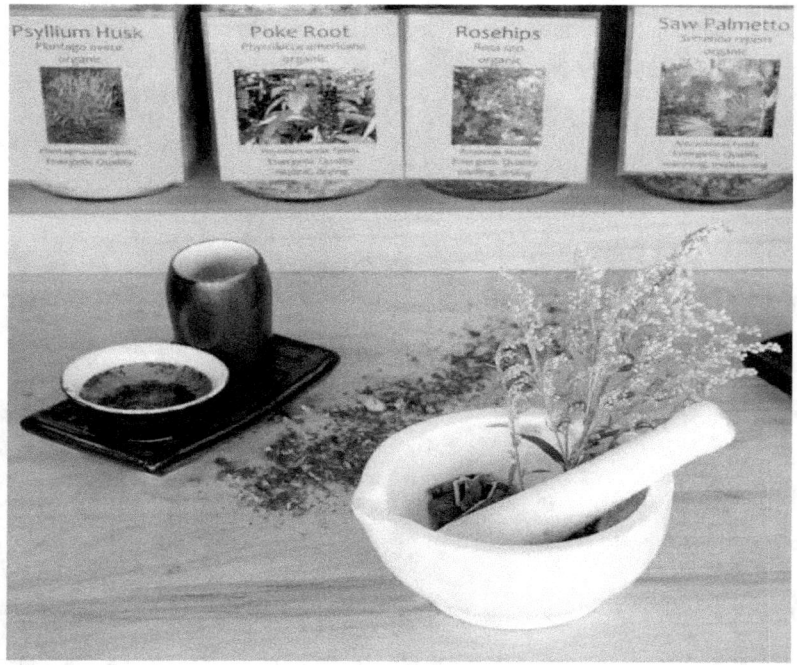

Before you start making your herbal remedies, you need to know all the different ways to make them. Here is a list which includes the shelf life of each.

● **Bolus**

This is a suppository and you can put it either in your rectum or your vagina, if you are female. These are generally made to directly apply the medicine to the affected area. This need to be used immediately.

How to make one:

In a double boiler add a tablespoon of coco butter and melt it. Add powdered herbs to the coco butter. Use aluminum to shape it into a bullet. Place it in the freezer to set. Insert the bolus and leave overnight.

- **Capsules**

This is the most common way for people to take remedies and supplements. These can keep their potency for up to two years.

To make them:

Mix the powdered herbs you wish to put in the capsules in a mixing bowl. Use a capsule making tool you can find online. Store them in a bottle with a tight lid in cool, dry place.

- **Compress**

This employs heat to help speed the healing properties of the ready to the injured area. They need to be used immediately.

How to make/use a compress:

Place 1/2 cup of herbs in a pot and three cups of water. Bring the water to a boil and simmer for an hour. Pour into a bowl and while still hot enough to place on the injured area, moisten a clean cloth and place on the injured area. As the compress cools change it out.

● **Decoction**

This is a type of tea which uses the roots, bark, and stems of the herb. For immediate use.

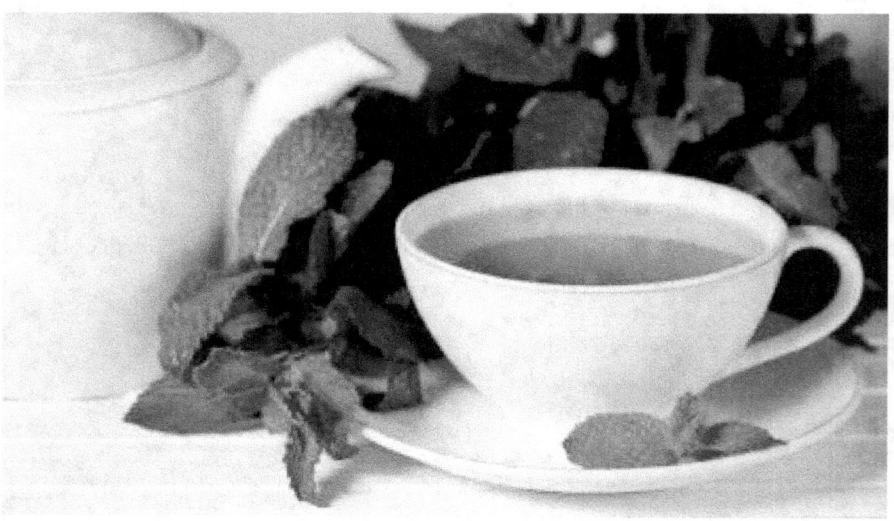

How to make one:

Therapeutic dose:

Use 1 tablespoon per each 6 ounce cup of water.

Maintenance dose:

Use 1 teaspoon per each 6 ounce cup of water.

Add the herbs to boiling water and boil for twenty minutes. Strain the plant matter out and add honey and lemon as needed.

• Extracts

This is a more potent preparation as far as this list is concerned. These are made by adding your herbs of choice to a solvent, letting the solvent leech the medicinal properties of herb out of the plant(s). You can either rub the extract on your skin or add up to 15 drops in a drink of your choice. Extracts last up to a year before losing potency.

How to make one:

You can use either four ounces of dried herbs or eight ounces of fresh, bruised (or mashed) herbs into a jar with a tight lid. Add to them one pint of either vinegar, alcohol, or rubbing alcohol. Shake the bottle twice a day for four days if the herbs you use are powdered or dry, and shake twice for fifteen days if you are using cut or whole fresh herbs.

• Hydrotherapy

This is an bath to which and strong herbal tea is added. This is commonly used for circulatory problems, skin problems, and to help detox.

How to make an herbal bath:

In a large stock pot, add one ounce of herbs. Fill the pot half-way. Bring the water to a boil and then simmer for twenty minutes. Strain out the herbs and add the tea to running water as you fill your bath.

• Infusion

This is a type of tea which uses the flowers and leaves of the herb.

To make an infusion:

Follow the directions for a decoction, but only boil for ten minutes.

• Oils

Herbal oils can be used both medicinally and for culinary purposes to add flavor to food. In herbal medicine, they are used for massage purposes.

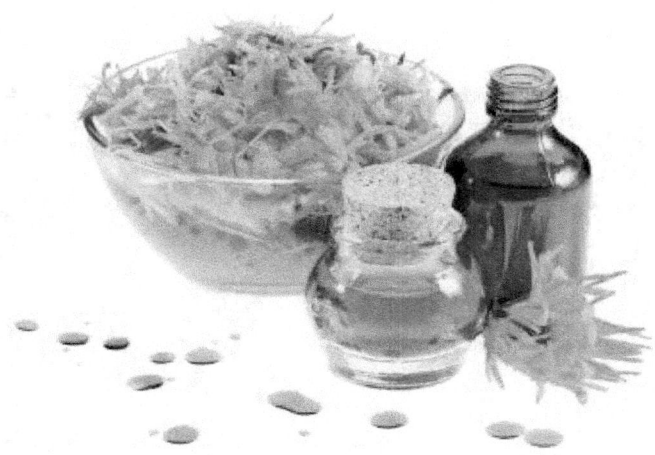

An herbal oil's shelf life is dependent on the oil you use to make it. Olive oil lasts the longest, but Sweet Almond is more commonly used and has a shelf life of six months to a year.

How to make an herbal oil:

Two ounces of an herb is added to one pint of oil. Sit the bottle, which should have a tight lid, in a warm place for four days. You can then strain the oil out for use. I quicker way of doing it is to use the same ratio and place the mixture into a crock pot on low overnight.

• Ointments

Ointments are thick and will stay on the skin for a longer period of time to help with minor injuries like bruises, bumps, sore muscles, and even rashes. They will keep for up to two years.

How to make an ointment:

You will need either Vaseline or non-petroleum jelly. Add two heaping tablespoons of the herbs to 1/2 a cup of the jelly. Heat on medium heat, stirring occasionally for twenty minutes. Strain the herbs out and place in a tightly lidded jar after it has cooled.

Poultices

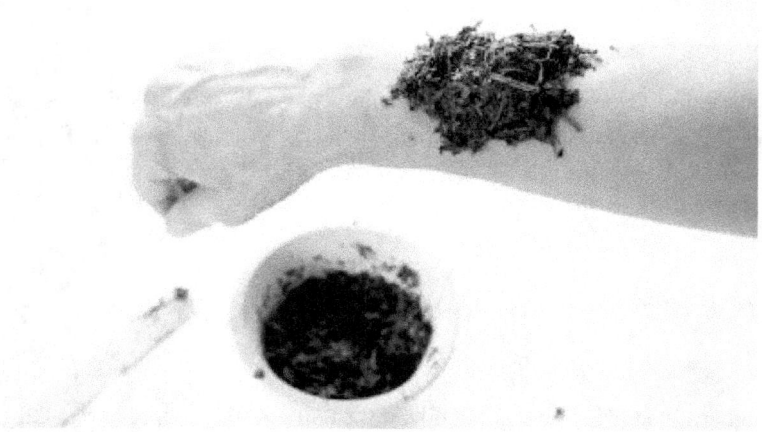

This is like a mask for your wound or injury. It is a thick mass of moistened herbs placed directly on the affected area. It is used in cases of bruising, insect bites, sprains and strains to keep the herbs in place for a long period of time. They can be applied either hot or cold but must be used as soon as they are made.

How to make a poultice:

Take an amount of herbs equal to the size of the area you wish to place the poultice. You can then mix in either hot water or herbal tea until it forms a thick paste. Powdered herbs are normally best for this. When it is still hot, but not hot enough to burn, place it on the affected area.

Powders

These are not commonly made it home due to a grinding process that can be tedious, but this is the preparation used in capsules, ointments at times, and also poultices.

Salves

These are like ointments because they are thick, but they are made completely different from their petroleum based counter part. Salves have a shelf life of about a year.

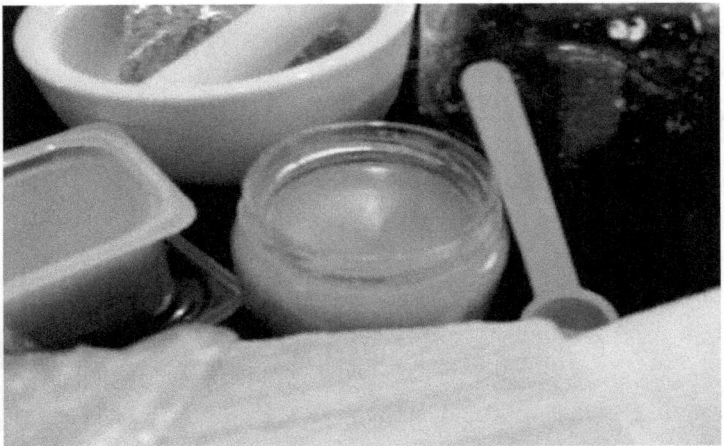

How to make salves:

You will need one cup of oil, 1/8 cup of beeswax beads and 1/4 cup of herbs. Make an herbal oil using the instructions for the crock pot. The next day, in a double boiler add the beeswax and melt. Stir in the oil without the herbs and place in a container with a tight lid. Apply to the affected area up to three times a day.

Syrups

These are good for stubborn colds, coughs, and even digestive problems. These keep for up to one week in the refrigerator.

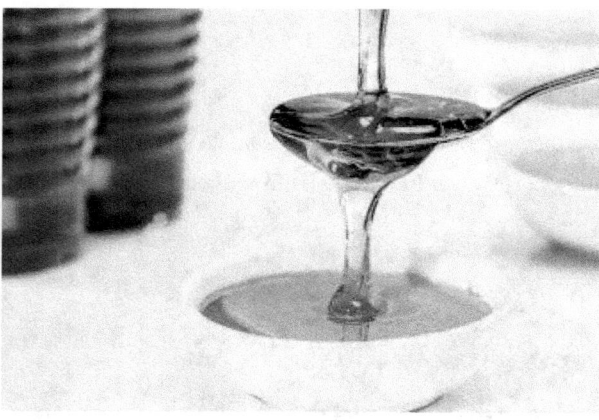

How to make a syrup:

Place 2 ounces of herbs in a stock pot and add one quart of water. Bring to a boil and let simmer until only a pint of water is left.

In a bottle or mixing container, place two ounces of either raw honey or vegetable glycerin. Strain out the herbs from the water and add the decoction to the honey or glycerin. Put a tight lid on it.

Tinctures

This are powerful concentrations of herbs made with alcohol in stead of water or vinegar. These are used in small doses and normally mixed in warm drinks for a more therapeutic kick. They can keep for up to two years.

How to make a tincture:

Add four ounces of herbals to a pint of either brandy or vodka. If you do not drink, you can add the herbs to boiled apple cider vinegar that has not been filtered. Allow the tincture to steep for up to four weeks, shaking every few days to mix the tincture well. You can strain out the herbs, but it is often not needed.

As you can see, there are a lot of ways to make and use herbs to treat injuries and illnesses. Which ones to make generally depend on the illness or injury and can be made using what you already have in your kitchen.

From a teacher to a mechanic, to do a job or hobby correctly, you need the proper tools. Making your own remedies is no different. Here is a list of what will be needed in order to make all the preparations above.

Glass or porcelain pots

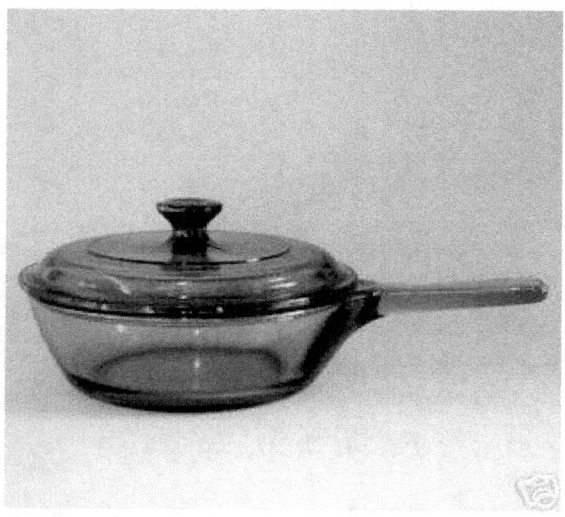

This may sound odd, but water and oil can leech the metal properties out of traditional pots and pans, often leading to a change in the way a preparation works. Glass and porcelain prevent the tainting of the mixtures.

Tea ball/reusable tea bags

These will often take a lot of the headache of straining herbs out for infusions, decoctions, syrups, and even herbal baths. You can find them online and even purchase one-use tea bags, both large and small, that you can use to keep your favorite blends. These can be sealed by using an iron or curling iron.

Double Boiler

You can also find these in glass. You can also rig your own by using a glass mixing bowl and placing it in a large pot that will hold it and add water to the pot. These are needed when you need to melt solid waxes and body butters without them touching the water.

Measuring spoons and cups

This are wonderful for measuring oils and herbs for smaller recipes.

Strainers

Plastic strainers are good for this, but you have to make sure the plastic won't shrink when you pour hot liquids through them.

Glass bottles and jars

You can find these online for reasonable prices, and they can be a life-saver for storing your preparations from salves to syrups and tinctures.

Food Scale

Make sure this measures in ounces to make it easier for larger preparations like herbal baths, syrups and the like.

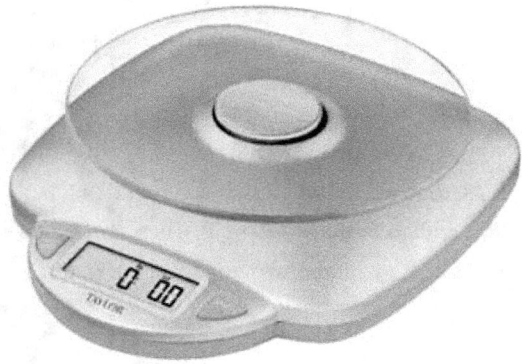

Crock Pot

Just about everyone has one in their home for all-in-one meals, but they are great for steeping herbs in oils to make the herbal oil process a lot faster.

Mixing spoons

These can be bamboo or silicone, but they are needed for mixing preparations and helping to place ointments and salves into their containers.

Labels

This may seem like a weird thing to put on a list for herbal preparations, but you need to label your preparations and add the expiration dates so you don't use something that's out-of-date.

Recipe book/box

This is key to keeping track of all the preparations you make on a regular basis.

Now, let's get onto the body systems and remedies.

Chapter 2 - The Structural System

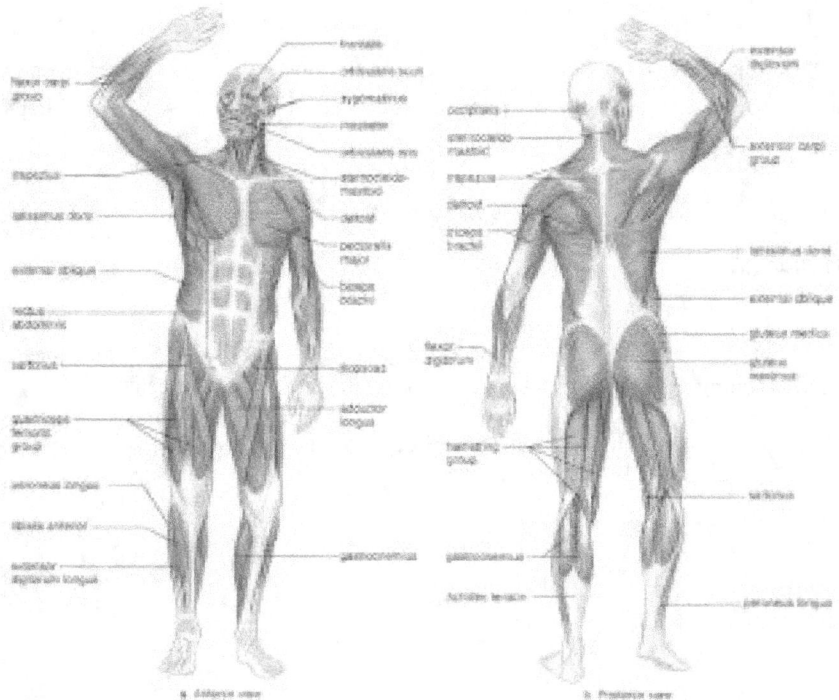

Your bones, joints, muscles, and skin all make up your structural system. Throughout our lives, depending on our activity level, we've all sprained an ankle, strained muscles, and even may have broken a bone. Most of us have had acne, but there are those of us who have had something we've tried to control but keep struggling with in terms of skin conditions.

Bruises

Everyday bumps and bruises can cause contusions, or bruises. There is a way to speed healing and get rid of the colorful reminder of having banged your body part.

Arthritis

This is a condition that attacks the joints and causes swelling, pain, and loss of movement/mobility. There are dietary restrictions to help prevent the swelling:

• Avoid the nightshade vegetables like tomatoes, potatoes, eggplant, and peppers.

• Keeping a diary of what you eat and how your arthritis reacts to what you eat can add to that list of foods to avoid.

Eczema and Psoriasis

These are skin conditions that are visible on the skin and can range from rashes that are cracked and bleeding to scale-like rashes that weep. Even though there are prescription medications that claim to bring these conditions under control, but they do it by suppressing the immune system, which can expose you to more serious diseases.

There are two ways to start being proactive when it comes to controlling these conditions:

• Get an allergy test. It have been proven, in some cases, these are allergic reactions to either environmental factors or food you eat.

• Manage your stress. This is easier said than done, but learning how to relieve and control stress will work wonders for controlling and, in some cases, relieve the condition altogether.

Bruise Salve

1 Cup of Sweet Almond oil (or Apricot Kernel oil if you're allergic to tree nuts)

1/8 Cup Beeswax

1 Tbsp *Arnica flowers*

(Really good for bruises)

1 Tbsp *Lavender Flowers*

(Good for Swelling)

(You can substitute Chamomile here)

1 Tbsp *Echinacea*

(Speeds healing)

Bruise poultice

2 Tbsp Arnica Flowers

Echinacea Tea

Joint Muscle Rub

6 Ounces of Sweet Almond Oil

2 Ounces of Olive Oil

2 Tbsp Juniper Berries

(Swelling and joint pain)

2 Tbsp Devil's Claw

(Joint pain and ligaments)

1 Tbsp Cinnamon

(Swelling and heating effect)

2 Tbsp Peppermint Leaves

(Cooling effect and anti-inflammatory)

Joint Herbal Bath

1/2 Ounce of Juniper Berries

1/2 Ounce of Lavender or Chamomile Flowers

Eczema Ointment

2 Tbsp Kelp

(Smooths the skin)

2 Tbsp Chamomile Flowers

(helps smooth skin)

2 Tbsp Echinacea

2 Tbsp Avocado Butter

(for extra moisture)

Psoriasis Rub

1/4 Cup Shea Butter

1/4 Cup Avocado Butter

(Both are excellent to toning and softening the skin and adding moisture)

2 Tbsp Lavender flowers

2 Tbsp Rose Petals

2 Tbsp Peppermint Leaves

1/4 ounce Aloe leaf

- Place the butters in a crock pot

- Add the herbs and steep overnight

- Strain out the herbs and place in a container with a tight lid.

- Let it cool before completely tightening the lid.

- Rub into the patches.

Chapter 3 - The Circulatory System

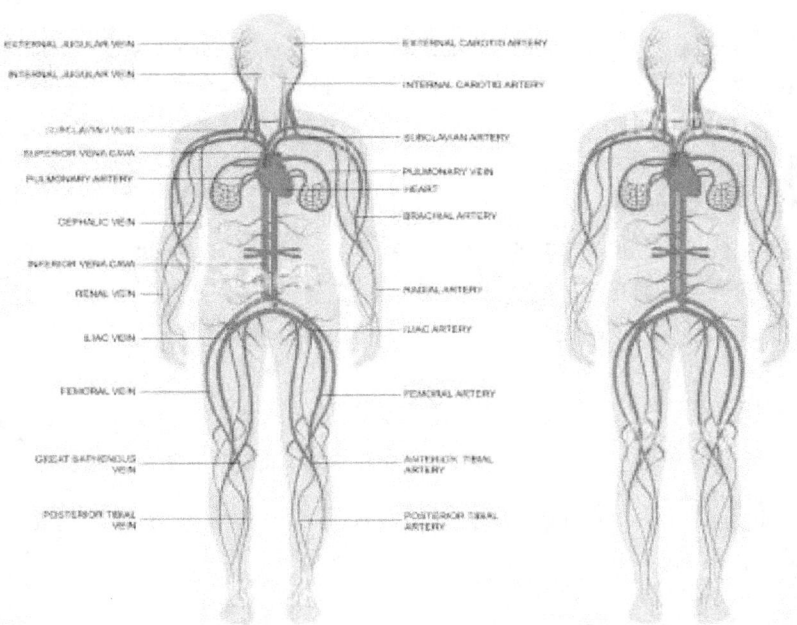

CIRCULATORY SYSTEM

Your heart and blood vessels are the carriers of the oxygen that leaves you lungs. They also help you convey vitamins, minerals, and amino acids to your muscles. When your blood vessels start to clog, you can experience shortness of breath, low energy, and put your heart at risk because it's trying to work harder to get the blood to where it needs to go.

Heart disease and hypertension are two of the most prominent problems in our society. Taking care of your heart is very important for a healthy life.

Hypertension

Simply put this is very high blood pressure on a regular/daily basis. Left untreated, it can lead to heart attack and stroke.

As the skin condition above, relieving and learning how to manage stress can help lower blood pressure.

Changes in diet can do this as well. Even walking three times a week for at least twenty minutes can reduce your blood pressure. Here are a couple of recipes that can help without interacting with any medications you may be taking.

For a Weak Heart

Some people are born with congenital heart disease or a weak heart. This leads to them tiring easily and being short of breath.

Infusion for weak valves

1 tsp hawthorn berries crushed

(Highly recommended for a weak heart)

1 tsp night blooming cereus

(for valve malfunctions)

1 tsp catnip (nervine)

Makes 1 therapeutic strength cup or 3 6-ounce regular strength cups.

Post-op Heart Attack Decoction

1 tsp hawthorn berries

1 tsp Dan Sheng Root

(Helps speed healing from heart operations)

1 tsp Lemon Zest (for flavor)

1 tsp Lavender flowers

(reduces swelling)

Hypertension

Just cooking with Basil and Cardamom can help to reduce your blood pressure. You can find these at any grocery store. Cooking with flaxseed is another way to help reduce your blood pressure.

Tea for Hypertension

Ginger tea is excellent for hypertension but if you can't handle the bite you can add Lavender and a little raw orange juice.

Blood Builders

These two recipes are to help strengthen blood vessels and for those who have low iron in their blood.

Iron Tea

1 tsp Red Raspberry leaves

1 tsp Red Clover flowers cut

1 tsp Butcher's Broom

Varicose Vein Bath

1/2 ounce Butcher's Broom

1/2 ounce Burdock Root

Chapter 4 - Digestive System

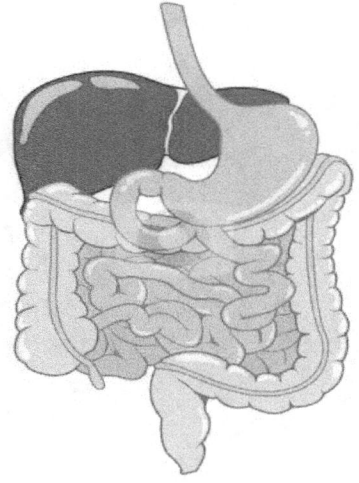

Upset stomachs, nausea, constipation, we've all experienced some sort of digestive issue. Stress, dietary choices, and even not getting enough fluids in your system on a daily basis can cause digestive issues. This does not discount actual intolerances, allergies, and diagnosed illnesses.

Heartburn

This is an over production of stomach acids to different degrees. Many antacids on the market can make this worse instead of better, leading to a complete dependence to the medication.

Here are some simple things you can do to help when it flares up:

• Parsley helps to curve heartburn. Chewing on a sprig will release the juice and stem the acid flow.

• Peppermint tea will help cool the burn.

Heartburn Tea

1 tsp Peppermint

(cools the core)

1 tsp Chamomile Flowers

1 tsp Lemon Balm leaves cut

(helps curve acid)

Drink cold

Marshmallow and Chamomile syrup

1 Ounce Marshmallow Root

(helps to absorb acids)

1 Ounce Chamomile Flowers

(calms the stomach)

2 Ounces Raw Honey

1 Tbsp every four to six hours.

Upset Stomach

This can be as small as an upset stomach to nausea and vomiting. Here are couple of things you can try:

- Chewing on a clove and swallowing the juice will alleviate nausea

- Putting a small amount of Allspice powder under your tongue will do the same.

Calming Tummy Tea

1 tsp Chamomile Flowers

1 tsp Peppermint leaves

1 tsp Fennel Seeds

(soothes the stomach)

Calming Tummy Syrup

1/2 ounce Peppermint Leaves

1/2 ounce Fennel Seeds

1/2 ounce Anise Seeds

1/2 ounce Lavender flowers

2 ounces raw honey

Chapter 5 - Nervous System

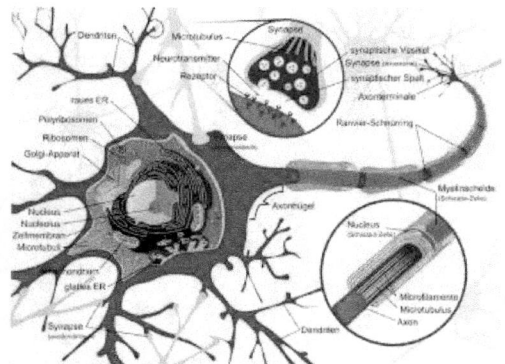

Made of our brain, eyes, spinal cord, and millions of synapses that fire off in order to deliver information to the brain the nervous system is truly a marvel, and many biologist have yet to unlock all its mysteries, but there are some ailments that are prevalent today which herbs to can help stem, if not help cure.

Alzheimer's Disease

Given a name in the late 80's this disease causes dementia in a patient, often reverting them back to child-like behavior and erasing memories of past experiences and even loved ones. There have been many reports of patients wandering off or family members getting in a car and driving only to not realize where they are.

Gingko Biloba has been tested, and in double blind studies has shown it can reverse early stages of Alzheimer's and lessen the severity of later stages.

Senility

This is quite different from dementia. Instead of wandering off or losing memories, it begins to present itself as being absent-minded and not able to recall things right away. This is simply due to the fact we need more B vitamins as we get older to help our brain function at the levels we are used to and for our nervous systems to function as they should.

Tea for concentration

1 tsp Peppermint leaves

1 tsp Gingko Bilboa

1 tsp Kelp (for B vitamins)

Extract for concentration

1 ounce Peppermint

1 ounce Kelp

1 ounce Gingko Biloba

1 ounce Gotu Kola

(Does the same thing as Gingko)

Anxiety

Anxiety can be debilitating. It can completely cripple someone leaving them unable to function. Here are couple of remedies that can help.

Nerve Tea

1 tsp Chamomile Flowers

1 tsp Catnip leaves

1 tsp Lavender Flowers

Herbal Bath

1/2 Ounce Lavender Flowers

1/2 Ounce Chamomile Flowers

Depression

Many people suffer from depression. It can take hours out of the day from your life by making you feel lethargic, and uninterested in everyday things. Just keep in mind, if you are bi-polar, you will have seek further advice from a licensed physician. The same goes for depression caused by chemical imbalances.

Saint John's Wort is the best herb to take for depression provided you are not already taking anti-depression medication.

Migraines

There are headaches that can be a nuisance and there are migraines that can make chunks of your absolutely miserable with a spike is driven through your head. Thought they are still trying to figure out all the root causes of migraines there are few things you can do to help stave some of them off:

• Log smells, foods and other things that can trigger a migraine.

• High stress can also cause migraines.

You can help relieve stress by meditation, and listening to soothing music when you come home from a busy day.

Migraine Tea

1 tsp Feverfew

1 tsp Peppermint

Chapter 6 - The Glandular System

This is the system that can regulate everything from the metabolism to you hormones and everything in between. Even though the liver is generally considered part of the digestive system, I have put it here because of it's filtering abilities and how it aids the pancreas in regulating blood sugar levels.

Diabetes

This is a well-known disease which involves the pancreas. Insulin is created by the pancreas to regulate blood sugar, but when starts to malfunction, it can produce less and less, leading to higher levels of glucose in the blood. This can cause dizziness and fainting spells, mood swings, and in more severe cases diabetic comas.

Nopal can help regulate glucose levels, and Stevia, a natural sweetener that is 10x sweeter than sugar, can as well.

Blood Sugar Tea

1 tsp Juniper Berries

1 tsp Ginger

1 tsp Billberry

Blood sugar Capsules

Equal parts of the following herbs in powder form:

Juniper berries

Nopal

Billberry

Stevia

It is recommended that you constantly check your blood sugar level if you are already on medication for this to make sure you are not lowering your glucose levels to dangerous numbers.

Liver/ Gall Bladder

Your liver and gall bladder take the brunt of the abuse when it comes to filtering out any toxins in your system. From fats to alcohol and even artificial additives, these two glands work hard to make sure you will not get ill from toxicity, but when they are overworked, you can run into problems.

Detox Tea

1 tsp Milk thistle seeds

(excellent for detoxing the liver)

1 tsp Dandelion root

(good for liver and water retention)

Prostate

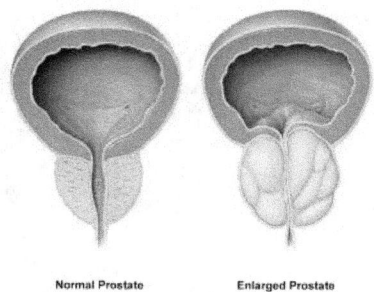

Normal Prostate   Enlarged Prostate

Prostate health is very important for men. Regular checks can lead to early detection for cancer and other prostate problems. There is also something you can take to maintain prostate health.

Saw Palmetto is the best supplement you take on a regular basis to maintain prostate health.

Menopause

The change of life can be hell on a woman. Here are a few suggestions you can try to make the transition to and the menopause itself easier.

Black Cohosh is the most popular, but it often does not work for all women.

Evening primrose can help with night sweats and hot flashes.

Wild Yam and Chaste Tree Berries are a wonderful combination for those that find the first two recommendations do work as well as they had hoped.

Chapter 7 - Keep Learning

There are a myriad more herbals out there than the ones I have mentioned in this book. Botanical.com is a great way to get started on your way to learning herbs. There are books which can continue your education as well. Today's Herbal, by Louise Tenney is a highly recommended start book for those wanting to learn more.

Experiment with different herbs and combinations to find what works best for you. You may even need to rotate supplements out from time to keep your body metabolizing different herbs and combinations. Your body can get used to them as time goes by.

Go onto online groups and forums to ask advice, learn about new herbs and expand your knowledge. You can even learn about essential oils and homeopathic remedies to compliment what you are already doing. You will be surprised what you can come up with when you have the right information and start mixing different herbs.

Conclusion

I hope this book answered questions that you had and didn't know you had. This book was meant to start you on your way to learning about a whole new field of natural health and taking control of your life, your body, and your health above all.

Please, be on the lookout for more books on natural health in this series, and as always, never stop asking questions.

www.ingramcontent.com/pod-product-compliance
Lightning Source LLC
Chambersburg PA
CBHW062016280526
45787CB00005B/2128